ADDITIONS TO CLASSICAL MATERIA MEDICA

NEW MEDICINES FROM Dr. CLARKE & HAHNEMANN

Compiled by

K.S. SRINIVASAN

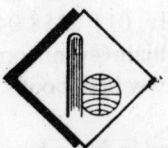

B. JAIN PUBLISHERS (P) LTD.

DELHI

Note from the Publishers

Any information given in this book is not intended to be taken as a replacement for medical advice. Any person with a condition requiring medical attention should consult a qualified practitioner or therapeutist.

Reprint Edition: 2003

All rights are reserved. No part of this book may be reproduced, stored in a retrieval system or transmitted, in any form or by any means, mechanical, photocopying, recording or otherwise, without any prior written permission of the author.

Price: Rs. 10.00

Published by: Kuldeep Jain for

B. Jain Publishers (P) Ltd.
1921, Street No. 10, Chuna Mandi,
Paharganj, New Delhi 110 055 (INDIA)
Phones: 2358 0800, 2358 1100, 2358 1300, 2358 3100
Fax: 011-2358 0471
Email: bjain@vsnl.com
Website: www.bjainbooks.com

Printed in India by:
**J.J. Offset Printers
522, FIE, Patpar Ganj, Delhi - 110 092**

ISBN 81-7021-663-X
BOOK CODE B-3531

PREFACE

The most complete records of provings and clinical symptoms available in print are TF Allen's *The Encyclopaedia of Pure Materia Medica (12 volumes)* and C Hering's *The Guiding Symptoms of Our Materia Medica (10 volumes)* published first in 1874 and 1879 respectively. Later Dr. JH Clarke published *A Dictionary of Practical Materia Medica (3 volumes)* in 1900.

Then on there is a yawning gap and no comparable records of provings and clinical symptoms came up because of many reasons, until Dr. O A Julian brought out his *Materia Medica of New Homoeopathic Remedies (1971)* in French which was later translated into English. There is also of course a publication of New Provings by James Stephenson prior to Julian's. Even now, we do not have a complete record of the provings being carried out in different parts of the world, published sporadically and lying scattered in journals. The need for compilation of all hitherto available reliable symptoms into one place is quite obvious.

During my re-reading of some of the old records of books and journals I came across additional material of value in respect of four remedies by Clarke and one by Hahnemann himself, which to the best of my knowledge have not so far been published in book form. Dr. Clarke had collected this material subsequent to the publication of his *Dictionary* and published them in the *"Homoeopathic World"* ; which were reprinted in the *"Homoeopathic Recorder"*. These are:

1. *Antimonium tartaricum*
2. *Antimonium sulphuratum aureum*
3. *Antimonium oxydatum*
4. *Antimonium natrum lacticum*

To these four by Dr. Clarke is added "Some Notes on *Badiaga* and Therapeutic Hints" of Hahnemann as 5th.

Attentive study of these would reveal the valuable gems in them, useful in day-to-day practice. The therapeutic range of *Ant-t.*, has become so wide, not just the 'rattlings', 'asphyxia', but Jaundice, Kala azar, sunstroke etc. It is also interesting that while Dr. H A Roberts and Dr. James Ward have included some symptoms in their 'Sensations As If', not all of the symptoms seem to have been included. In the Synthetic Repertory I have not found some of the symptoms; for example "MIND, Despairs of recovery"; "Unusual wild gaiety, towards evening"; both of which Clarke has given in italics; also "child clings to nurse and calls for help with cough".

With regard to Hahnemann's observations and his Notes on *Badiaga* need anyone say that they are pure gold ?

December 1989   K S SRINIVASAN

INDEX

		PAGES
1.	SOME THERAPEUTIC HINTS AND NOTES ON BADIAGA *by Samuel Hahnemann*	1
2.	ANTIMONIUM NATRUM LACTICUM *by J. H. Clarke*	3
3.	ANTIMONIUM SUPHPURATUM AUREUM *by J.H. Clarke*	6
4.	ANTIMONIUM OXYDATUM *by J.H. Clarke*	11
5.	ANTIMONIUM TARTARICUM *by J.H. Clarke*	15

SOME THERAPEUTIC HINTS OF HAHNEMANN AND HIS NOTES ON BADIAGA

The Homoeopathic World, Vol. LXII, Dec. 1927, pp. 309-336 contained some 'Notes and Translations from French and German Hahnemann Documents in the possession of Mr. Mazzini Stuart'. Some extracts from this was published in the *Homoeopathic Recorder*, Feb.15, 1928. This contained some therapeutic hints of Hahnemann; his views on the eradication of hereditary psora; and also his Notes on *Badiaga*.

"An extract from a letter of Hahnemann's to von Boenninghausen, on bone abscesses, written in Paris, Oct. 23, 1840: I do not deny that in bone abscesses as a rule cure only takes place with difficulty. *Angus.* has sometimes been useful. To me they seem to be of a two-fold nature, of which one kind seems to need remedies of a basic nature, such as *Calc.*, *Hepar sulph. calc.*, the other kind needs acids such as *Acid nitric*, *Silicea* and *Acid phos*. Of the latter you have an indication (in, I believe, 613, *Acid phos*. of the 2nd edition of *Chronic Diseases*) *Asaf.* has rarely been of any use to me. *Cuprum* and *Angus*, must also be taken into consideration. In very weak constitutions *Arn.* must not be forgotten. In Tinea, proemisis proemittendis, *Staph.* has rarely failed me, particularly in very high dynamisations. To inquire if they have been infected with itch is a useless proceeding. One is only told half the truth. Apart from this hereditary Psora cannot be denied".

The next translation is a fragment of one of Hahnemann's letters:

"Probably, if with the first pregnancy, during the time of pregnancy the antipsoric treatment were properly carried out, one might succeed in freeing mankind from the evil of hereditary psora, a success of far greater value than the eradication of smallpox by vaccination".

Mrs. Wheeler (who translated Dr. Haehl's life of Hahnemann) ends with a translation of Hahnemann's notes on *Badiaga*:

"With emotional excitement violent palpitation with joyous sensation, lasting one minute.

Frequent stools, diarrhoea on the first day.

Nervous Excitement.

Impatience.

Burning and itching behind the ears.

A chain of swollen glands in the neck.

The last joints of the ring finger swollen and painful.

(At the side of notepaper Hahnemann makes the following remark: dry SCAB between fingers).

Irritability.

Peevishness.

Nausea as at the beginning of sea-sickness.

Early morning, twice urinating; much urine, afterward frequent desire to urinate and yet only a few drops pass accompanied with severe pain in the arms.

During the day frequent heat waves in the face with some (word illegible).

Feeling as if the hair was standing up on the head.

Vertigo, stupefaction to the point of reeling about in the evening when going to lie down.

Pressive pain in the forehead.

Light and noise annoy her.

Slow digestion--enormous quantity of flatulence is eructated.

Strong sexual excitement for two weeks.

After being heated through climbing mountains, tremor, restlessness, anxiousness, quick breathing.

Hard skin on soles of feet.

Itching on soles of feet.

After speaking loudly, stitch under left nipple.

Burnig stitches in the forehead, temples and eye sockets.

Pressure in the region of the stomach when sitting bent which disappears on sitting upright.

Itching over the whole body as if flea-bitten, increasing towards evening and worse in bed.

When walking in the open-air a feeling of tiredness in the upper thigh".

ANTIMONIUM NATRUM LACTICUM
(Ant. n.l.)*

J. H. CLARKE, M.D.

Double Lactate of Antimony and Soda. Sodium Antimonyl Lactate. Sb $(C_3 H_5 O_3)_3$. $Na_2(C_3 H_5 O_3)_3$. Solution.

Clinical—Debility. Diarrhoea. Heart, weakness of; palpitation of. Hydrogenoid constitution. Indigestion. Jaundice. Skin, affections of.

Characteristics—Dr. F.B. Percy records in N.E.M.G., December, 1901, an involuntary proving of *Ant. n.l.* communicated to him by a correspondent who himself was poisoned whilst manufacturing it for dyeing purposes. Powdered metallic antimony is dissolved in a mixture of lactic and nitric acids. The nitric acid is used to convert the metal into an oxide, soluble in lactic acid. When the nitric acid is used up, one-half of the remaining lactic acid is neutralized with soda. "The double lactate of antimony and soda is a hygroscopic, non-crystallisable salt, which is absorbed through the skin with great readiness. Shortly after beginning the manufacture of this", says Dr. Percy's correspondent, "I noticed a decided lowering of the general health with great *sensitiveness to cold*. I was only comfortable in a room at 80 to 85 degrees, and was *obliged to give up cold baths*, to which I was regularly accustomed up to this time. There was also great digestive disturbance, much gas in the intestines, watery and mucous discharges from the intestines, but no pain, and a nasty coated tongue, torpid liver, and yellow skin. The whites of the eyes showed yellow as well. The heart, which had always been quick but strong, became most erratic, jumping from fifty-six to a hundred and fifty beats per minute, and from weak to strong and *vice versa*. The mental disturbance was more pronounced than the physical. An extreme listlessness was accompanied with the most extreme melancholy. The thing which finally led me to the cause of the trouble was the breaking out of watery pustules on the wrists and arms, principally an intense itching of the inflamed parts. The pustules resembled *Rhus* poisoning". "Soda and a tonic" was prescribed by a physician but without effect. Then iodide of potassium, in one to one solution, five drops thrice

---

*Repr. from The Homeopathic World, 1928, LXIII, 326. This article is one of the supplementary articles to the Dictionary of Materia Medica. Antim. nat. lact. is new to the materia medica and does not appear in the Dictionary itself. -J. H. C.

daily, gave immediate relief. Nitroglycerine relieved the heart symptoms. Five months after the poisoning, though nearly normal, the prover was still unable to resume his cold baths, and was still more or less dependent on nitroglycerine.

Nearly all the above effects are paralleled in *Ant. c.*, but the wrist as special locus of the eruption is peculiar, and the action on the heart is more pronounced. The hygroscopic nature of the salt should be noted in connection with the extreme sensitiveness to cold it produces. It is evidently a powerful "hydrogenoid". The > in a warm room is a point of difference from *Ant.c.* < cold bathing is characteristic in both.

Relations—*Antidoted by Kali iod.* (general symptoms, weakness, mental depression); *Glon.* (heart symptoms). *Compare Rhus, Merc., Psor.,* (eruption on wrists)

SYMPTOMS

1. MIND

    Extreme listlessness accompanied by extreme melancholy.

3. EYES

    White of eyes yellow.

8. MOUTH

    Coated tongue.

11. STOMACH

    Great digestive disturbance.

12. ABDOMEN

    Much gas. "Torpid liver".

13. STOOL

    Watery and mucous stools.

19. HEART

    Pulse most erratic; jumping from 56-150 and from weak to strong and *vice versa*.

22. UPPER LIMBS

    Eruption of watery pustules on wrists and arms with intense itching of inflamed parts.

24. GENERALITIES

Decided lowering of general health.
Extreme sensitiveness to cold; only comfortable in a room at 80—85 degrees--compelled to give up cold baths.

25. SKIN

Yellow.
Watery pustules on wrists and arms; an intense itching of inflamed parts.

[From "THE HOMOEOPATHIC RECORDER" Feb. 15, 1929 Pages : 84 - 85.]

ANTIMONIUM SULPHURATUM AUREUM (Ant. s. a.)*

J. H. CLARKE, M.D.

Clinical— Bronchitis, pains in. Cough: of influenza. Headache. Hip joint, affections of. Laryngitis. Rheumatism. Shoulders, affections of.

Characteristics— Ant. s.a. was introduced into medicine by Glauber in 1654; was proved by Mayrhoffer in 1845, and the proving was published by Buchner in 1874. My chief clinical guide to the use of this remedy is H. Goullon, whose article may be found in *The Homoeopathic World*, January 1902, entitled *"Tips for Allopaths Who Really Want to Know"*. It is copied from *H. Encyc.*, which gives a translation of the article as it appeared in *Leipziger Pop. Zeit. f. Hom.*, October, 1901. Goullon says :

At the conclusion of an acute laryngeal or bronchial catarrh, or even in the acute form of this ailment, and even in chronic catarrh of the aerial passages, this is a glorious remedy with an effect frequently wonderful. It lessens the cough so beautifully, and the coarse, hoarse voice regains its timbre. It cannot, indeed, take the place of *Spo., Bro.* and *Phos.*; these have their own sphere of action; but if such a "cougher"-excuse the word-comes along who finds no rest from coughing, either day or night, while his throat and chest are *sore from coughing*, he must quickly get Ant. s. a., 1 trit., three or four times a day and also at night, as much as would lie on the point of a penknife.

This I have verified many times. The indication *sore from coughing* is one of the best keynotes I know in the materia medica. It has helped me with numberless cases of influenza cough, in grain doses of the 3rd trit. It is a clinical observation or inference, as is Hering's "Hard, dry cough, no expectoration". There are, however, these symptoms in the proving: "Tickling as from mucus with inability to expectorate. Pressure and constriction in the bronchial tubes. Bronchi full with difficult respiration. Increased mucous expectoration mixed with blood, of a sweetish taste." The *sensitiveness of the bronchi* is peculiar; and there is also sensitiveness of other parts, as surface of abdomen, scrotum. "Fulness" and "tension" and "pressure" run through the proving.

---

* Supplementary to the D.M.M. in which this does not appear.

There are also burning pains. The < from washing of the other *Antimonies* appears in *Bleeding of the nose from washing*. There is < also after sleep (headache; pains in thorax and spine). Among localities affected are: hip-joints and groins; shoulder-joint (l); bones of forearm; posterior nares and throat ("plug" sensation, as *Ant. c.*); umbilicus; scrotum (eruption like *Ant. o.*).

SYMPTOMS

1. MIND

   Apprehensiveness with heaviness in praecordium.

2. HEAD

   Head confused; from severe injury in abdomen.
   Forehead confused.
   Pressive headache.
   Headache in forepart.
   One-sided headache, especially l. temporal region. *Burning in the head*; with eye complaints.
   Wakes after midnight with dull headache after dreamy sleep.

4. EARS

   Reddish swelling behind r. ear, leaving a redness and scurfiness.

5. NOSE

   Violent coryza with loss of smell.
   Catarrh and fluent coryza with impeded respiration (morning), confused head and impaired appetite.

7. TEETH

   Pressing, boring, tearing boothache.

8. MOUTH

   Much saliva and water collected in the mouth. Tongue very thickly coated yellow; slimy with pasty taste.

9. THROAT

   Increased mucus from back of throat.
   Burning and heat in the fauces.
   Pressure and tensive feeling in the throat, especially at larynx.
   SORENESS OF THROAT AND CHEST FROM COUGHING. (Goullon).

10. APPETITE

Pasty taste.
Taste sweetish, bitter and flat.
Loss of appetite, almost a loathing of food.
Appetite increased to decided hunger.

11. STOMACH

Pressure and fulness in stomach and stomach-pit.
Burning, sticking sensation in whole l. side, especially of l. lumber muscles.
Abdomen tense, full.
Twisting in intestines.
Great sensitiveness of intestine and colon; especially at anus.
Tensive drawing pains in groins.

13. STOOL AND ANUS

Constipation, with tenesmus and burning pains in anus.

14. URINARY ORGANS

In urethra, tickling with increased urine.
Increased urine with much tickling and tensive sensation in penis.
Urine increased, dark red (containing traces of antimony after 6 grains).

15. MALE SEXUAL ORGANS

Itching and eruption on scrotum extends to perineum.
Sexual desire unusually excited.
Extraordinary sensitiveness of genitals.

17. RESPIRATORY ORGANS

Pressure and tensive feeling in throat, specially at larynx.
Tickling as from mucus in larynx and air passages; with inability to expectorate.
Bronchi feel full with *difficult respiration. No rest from coughing day or night*, THROAT AND CHEST SORE FROM COUGHING. (Goullon).

18. CHEST

Heaviness in praecordium and apprehensiveness. SORENESS OF CHEST, from cough (Goullon).
Rheumatic pains over whole thorax and spine with difficult, noisy inspiration, on sudden waking after midnight.

19. HEART

    Heaviness in praecordium and apprehensiveness.
    Pulse soft; small, suppressed.

20. NECK AND BACK

    Tensive, pressing feeling in cervical vertebrae, neck and ribs.
    Burning, sticking sensation in l. lumbar muscles and whole l. side.

21. LIMBS

    Tensive feeling on muscles of sholders and thighs.
    Stiff tensive pains in.
    Stiff tensive pains in joints, mornings.
    Constant drawing, tearing, rheumatic pains in joints.
    Itching of hands and feet.

22. UPPER LIMBS

    Arms heavy in morning.
    Painful immobility of l. arm.
    Rheumatic pains in joints of arms.
    Boring, tearing in joints of arms and hand.
    Pressive tensive pain in l. shoulder-joint.
    Twitching like electric shocks through both ulnar nerves, especially in elbow-joint.
    Pressure and heaviness in bones of forearm.
    Swelling of fingers.
    Tensive swollen feeling of fingers.

23. LOWER LIMBS

    Pustules, elevated, dry, on inner surface of thighs, itch, feel tense, pain on walking and involve the whole leg in sympathy; remain three weeks, then dry and desquamate.
    Heaviness and weariness.
    Tensive and rheumatic trouble in hip-joint and groin.
    Slight swelling of knee and ankle.

24. GENERALITIES

    Sense of great weakness and prostration in morning.

25. SKIN

    Itching, especially of scrotum and inner surface of thighs.
    Pustules.

26. **SLEEP**

Vivid dreams and sudden waking after midnight with restlessness, rheumatic pains over whole thorax and spine; dyspnoea.
Sleep with dreaming, with sudden waking.
Deep, sleep with sweat.
Heavy, unrefreshing sleep.

27. **FEVER**

General chilliness with shivering down whole spine.
Chills alternate with heat.
Moderate sweat at night.

[From "THE HOMOEOPATHIC RECORDER" Feb. 15, 1929 *Pages* : 258 – 260]

ANTIMONIUM OXYDATUM (Ant. o)*

J. H. CLARKE, M.D.

SESQUIOXIDE OF ANTIMONY $SB_2 O_3$
TRITURATION

Clinical : Acne. Boils. Debility. Dysuria. Glands enlarged. Gonorrhoea. Impotence. Night sweats. Perspiration, excessive. Prostate, affections of. Pustules. Testes, atrophy of. Urine, disorder of.

Characteristics : The symptoms of *Ant. o.* have been obtained from the effect of the fumes in antimony works. The record is in Allen's Encyclopaedia obtained from *Alg. Hom. Zeit.* 20, 122, and *Rev. de la Med. Hom.* 2, 194. The head, chest and urogenital organs were chiefly affected and a complete relaxation of the whole organism with depression. Pustular eruptions were also well marked. Probably in *Ant. o.* we have the purest antimony effects of all the antimony provings. The chief localities are the same in all, but *Ant. o.* has more pronounced action on the genito-urinary system than the others, producing dysuria, strangury and gonorrhoea-like discharge, impotence and atrophy of penis and testes. In the head there are lightning-like pains from front to back; occipital pains; and pains behind the glabella. Stitches prevail in the chest. There is extreme weakness, depression, restlessness and profuse sweat.

Ant. ox. enters into the compositions of "James' Fever Powders", a famous remedy of long ago, which consists of one part of *Ant. ox.* to two parts of Calcium phosphate.

Relations : Compare *Ant. l.* Red urine, *Oc. c.* Impotence, *Lyc.* Pains in head from before backward, *Anac., Bell., Bry., Naja., Nux.,* Sleepiness with headche, *Gels., Lach., Puls.* Difficult tenacious expectoration, *K. bi.*

xxx

---

*Repr. from The Homeopathic World, LXIV, Jan. 1929, p.12, supplement † The Dictionary of Materia Medica, in which this does not appear.

SYMPTOMS

1. **MIND**

   Depression and general relaxation.

2. **HEAD**

   Violent headache; with tearing in limbs.
   Slight headache increasing to intolerable degree.
   Continuous fatiguing pain immediately behind the glabella.
   Lightning-like stitches from front to back, disappearing suddenly but leaving frontal headache.
   Stitches and burning in occiput and nape.
   Violent stupefying pain in occiput, worse evenings, so exhausting he falls into unrefreshing sleep.

8. **MOUTH**

   Tongue coated white.

10. **APPETITE**

    Diminished or lost.

12. **ABDOMEN**

    Distended with incarcerated flatus.
    Colic, without diarrhoea.

13. **STOOL AND ANUS**

    Diarrhoea; troublesome, frequent, with griping, consisting of food evacuated soon after eating.

14. **UNINARY ORGANS**

    Indescribable lameness in urinary apparatus.
    Pains and urging at neck of bladder and burning in urethra during urination.
    Discharge of a few drops of mucus from urethra.
    Gonorhoea-like discharge from urethra.
    Painful discharge of urine, *guttation*.
    Dysuria with mucous discharge causing burning in urethra.
    Strangury.
    Urine, deep orange-yellow, almost red.

Addition to Classical Materia Medica 13

Deep-red and bloody urine, causing burning in urethra, a whitish mucus exuding after urine ceased.

15. **MALE SEXUAL ORGANS**

    Atrophy of penis and testes.
    Penis flaccid.
    Loss of feeling and sexual appetite.
    Impotence.
    Burning in glans.
    Pain in testes.
    Pustules thick on genitals.

17. **RESPIRATORY ORGANS**

    Cough; violent, shattering, dry, with stitches in chest; dry, painful, ending in difficult expectoration of tenacious mucus.
    Respiration difficult, with sibilant rales all over chest.

18. **CHEST**

    Very great constriction, with stitches.
    Oppression, constriction and irritation to cough.
    Lancination along edge of ribs and in neck.
    Sharp stitches through chest to shoulders and back.
    Violent stitches with dry cough.

20. **NECK AND BACK**

    Swelling of cervical glands.
    Sensitive pains in loins.
    Sharp pains in sacro-lumbar regions.
    Pustules on neck and body.

21. **LIMBS**

    Pain in all the limbs.
    Spasms.
    Pustules on nates; bends of limbs; on thighs and scrotum.

24. **GENERALITIES**

    Weakness and relaxation of the whole organism.
    Excessive general irritability.
    Great sensitiveness.

25. **SKIN**

    Pustular eruption like pocks on body generally, esp. neck, lower abdomen, genitals, bends of limbs.

26. **SLEEP**

   Restlessness preventing sleep.
   Sleeplessness.
   Dreams, fatiguing, anxious; frequent starting.

27. **FEVER**

   Of intermittent type.
   Prespiration; profuse with general weakness; debilitating during sleep; tormenting, pouring sweats every time after sleep, followed by great exhaustion.
   Excessive night sweats.

   [From "THE HOMOEOPATHIC RECORDER" Feb. 15, 1929
   Pages : 185 – 186]

ANTIMONIUM TARTARICUM (Ant. t.)*

J.H. CLARKE, M.D.

Clinical — Jaundice, Kala-Azar. Lumbrici. Lungs, oedema of. Pregnancy, salivation of. Tonsils enlarged. Sunstroke.

Characteristics — [Errata : p. 129, l. 12 from bottom for "exception" *read* "Eruption"; p. 130, l. 8. from bottom for "Mild" *read* "Wild".] *Ant. t.*, says Hering, is "An invention of the Alchemists, very popular with them, forbidden by the French Academy, finally introduced and much used and abused by the old school. Proved by Hahnemann and some of his students, it was published by Stapf in 1844". This is undoubtedly the most active of the antimonial preparations and has been the agent used in many cases of criminal poisoning. Three recent instances of the latter are recorded in B.M.J., April 11, 1903. The autopsies in each case revealed the same state of things: the body in a remarkable state of preservation, in one case nearly two years after death; the tissues were dry and drained of fluid; there were signs of gastroenteritis without ulceration. The symptoms of two of the cases are contributed by Dr. J.M. Sliker, who attended. They were those of persistent vomiting and diarrhoea; but in one case, that of a young woman, aged 19, there was a symptom which shows the tetanising properties of *Ant. t.* as well as the centering of its action on the stomach. (The autopsy in this case revealed "dark rings round the sunken eyes".) "About the sixth day", says Dr. Sliker, "I noticed spasm of the muscles and rigidity. The spasms were ushered in by pain in the rectum"; [the rectal pain was apprently set up in the first place by attempts at rectal feeding, the patient being unable to retain the injections or nutrient enules] "then the muscles of the abdomen became rigid. From this the rigidity extended to the legs and then to the upper extremities. The same order was observed in each attack, the abdominal muscles being first affected and so on. They occurred independently of the vomiting. On one occasion the muscular spasms came on as I was palpating the abdomen, and I could distinctly feel the muscles contract under my hand. Morphine suppositories seemed to possess a strong controlling influence on them." This is paralleled by a symptom in Allen from another poisoning case, the effect of 2 drachms, "constant contraction of

---

* Repr. from the Homoeopathic World, Apr. and Jun., 1929, p. 96. supplement to article in the D.M.M.

all the muscles, especially of abdomen and upper extremities"; and also by symptoms of Hahnemann's. "He had scarcely fallen asleep when he was seized with electric shocks and jerks all of which came from the abdomen; it threw now one arm, now another, away from the body; now a foot; now it threw the whole body into the air". Another point in the antimony effect brought out by Dr. Sliker's cases is the intense debility of *Ant. t.* Although the patients were severely ill the doctor was astonished in each case when he heard they were dead; there was sudden collapse in syncope. In both cases there was general abdominal tenderness, most marked in the epigastrium. Kent (*J. of Hcs.*, March, 1901) lays stress on the facial expression of *Ant. t.* as characterizing the particular quality of its debility. Face pale, sickly, eyes sunken with dark rings round them, lips pale and shrivelled, nostrils dilated and flapping rapidly, dark, sooty appearance inside; cold sweat on the pale or blue face. This condition of debility occurs in *catarrhal* states in the later stages when weakened by the force of the acute disease, or in such affections occuring in patients already enfeebled, or in very young or very old patients. Old *gouty* patients, always shivering, pale and with enlarged joints." Every spell of wet weather brings on catarrh of the chest with copious secretion. Children who have frequent attacks of bronchitis from cold wet weather, constantly recurring with rattling in the chest; chilly and pale, (*Florid* children who do not look ill when they have colds and rattling in the chest and are not prostrated require *K. sul.*) A relaxed passive condition is Kent's description of the *Ant. t.* debility. It corresponds to the catarrh of old drunkards with rattles in the chest. There is an awful anxiety in the stomach. A dropsical condition of the tissues and joints is also antim. effect. Kent has seen this produced in horses by excessive dosing with *Ant. c.*

In old times *Ant. t.* was the universal remedy in cases of pneumonia and this, like all routine practice, led to disastrous results. But there was, as usual, truth at the bottom of the treatment. Goullon has had great success with *Ant. t.* 1 trit. in 5 grain doses, and commends the practice for trial to allopaths "who really want to know". Stonham (*B.H.J.*, April, 1912) quotes a case from Dudgeon illustrating what *Ant. t.* can do in a case *in extremis*. An old lady had been taken ill and had been under the care of an eminent practitioner and two baronets. She was sinking fast, and as a last resort the friends decided to try homoeopathy and sent for Dr. Dudgeon, who found her perfectly insensible, pulse 140 and intermittent; tongue black; and she had a bed-sore as big as a soup plate. Dudgeon told the friends that he did not think the patient had fortyeight hours to live, but he gave *Ant. t.* and occasional doses of *Phos.*, and she recovered completely. Stonham gives a gastro-intestinal case from Dr. Dyce Brown which is quite to the point: Mrs. H-was taken ill on July 1, 1876, with shivering, followed by fever, severe vomiting and purging. Under allopathy she was getting worse and Dyce Brown was called in on July 5. He found the patient with an extremely rapid pulse constantly sick, the vomiting having now been replaced by empty retching. Nausea constant. Even a mouthful of cold water was at once rejected, although she was tormented with great thirst. Profuse watery diarrhoea; stools too frequent to count. Marked abdominal tenderness. Tongue coated from tip to back with a thick white, smooth, creamy coat, the edges being red. *Acon.* tincture 5 drops in three quarters of a tumbler of water, and *Ant. t.* 1 x, 2 grains in another tumbler, a teaspoonful of each every alternate hour. Next day, pulse normal, skin moist and cool, retching stopped and only occasional nausea; tongue almost clear; the feeling in the abdomen was soreness rather than pain. *Ant. t.* given alone rapidly completed recovery. Stonham quotes from Dr. Nichol a case of small-pox in which *Ant. t.* revealed its action. J.T., 28, strong never vaccinated, contracted small-pox. Violent chills were followed by high fever with restlessness, nausea and malaise. The chills seemed to originate in the region of the spine, spreading over the trunk of the body and always from within outward. Patient stupid and drowsy. Dull headache with pressure on brain and occasional delirium. Thickly coated tongue, with bitter sickening taste. Mouth and throat filled with pocks. Nausea and vomiting always followed by prostration and clammy skin and feeble pulse. Swelling of abdomen with rumbling and gurgling but no diarrhoea. A marked bronchitis was present from the commencement, gradually extending to the lungs, as catarrhal pneumonia with very copious secretions. The eruption was so thick and continuous that the patient seemed as if he was smeared from head to foot with honeycomb. *Ant. t.*, 3x, unaided, brought about complete recovery with only a few traces of pockmarks on the nose. Dudgeon records two skin cases illustrating *Ant. t. localities.* (1) A young lady, 18, had for 7 months a disagreeable eruption on her face – small pimples filled with matter, not much larger than a pin's head, extending from the roots of the hair down centre of forehead to tip of nose. She had been under an eminent skin specialist without benefit. *Ant. t.* 1x, one grain in 3 ounces of water, a tablespoonful twice daily cured in a fortnight. (2) A young lady, 16, had for upwards of a year a disfiguring eruption on the face, consisting of small discrete pustules, which, after drying up, left for a long time an ugly bluish red mark,, so that her naturally handsome features were quite spoilt by the blotches left by the old pustules as well as by the yellow-headed moist pimples. All parts of the face were affected, nose, forehead, cheeks and chin. In addition, for upwards of a month she had been tormented with a similar eruption about the genitals and tops of the thighs, which was so excessively painful that she could not sit down without suffering and was quite unable to walk even a few hundred yards. She was unable to sleep for the pain and irritation and lost her strength, spirits and appetite. *Ant. t.* 2x, gr. 1, in 9 tablespoonfuls of water, a spoonful three times a day. There was immediate general improvement. In a fortnight the eruption was quite gone from the genitals; and in three weeks only a trace was left about the chin and nose, and another week those had gone too. Dr. Stonham concludes his article with an eye case. Dr. Casanova contracted granular ophthalmia by unconsciously rubbing his eyelids after examining a patient. Acute conjunctivitis with granulation on the lids followed. The lids became thickened, sight impaired, with burning and itching in eyebrows and lids, and crusty formations on the edges of the lids during the night, <reading, cold air, stimulants. This lasted three years. He then tried a lotion of *Ant. t.* gr. ii in 3ii of distilled water and used as a lotion twice a day. It caused a good deal of smarting, but at the end of two weeks the granulating had diminished considerably and the sight was much improved. After two more weeks there were no more vestiges of granulation. The lotion was continued, more attenuated for two months when the eyes and sight were normal. Dr. O.M. Drake (quoted A.H., Dec. 15, 1895 from H.P.) related a case of sunstroke which came under his care in October, 1876, the attack having occurred in the previous July, the patient having been under allopathic treatment in the meantime. *Lyc.* was selected as the remedy best indicated, and under this in the 200th he made some progress, being enabled to go out, though unfit for work. The potency of the remedy was changed up and down, but no further progress was made. One day Drake noticed the patient repeatedly pass his hand downward from the forehead over the nose as if to brush something off. Questioned about it he said that for a long time he had had a *feeling over the bridge of his nose as though a horse hair were drawn tightly across it*, and every little while he found himself trying to remove it. Occasionally he had the sensation of having spectacles on, the bows pressing unpleasantly on the back of the ears. This feeling he was unable to brush away. *Ant. t.* 200 was given, and in three weeks the man was well and able to return to his work. This is noteworthy among the *Peculiar Symptoms* of *Ant. t.* Others are : sensation as of a small leaf obstructing the

Addition to Classical Materia Medica

larynx. Lower jaw-joints as if dislocated. Oesophagus sore and sensitive. Headache extending to root of nose. As of tight band across forehead. As if the brain were put together in lumps. Pain from neck over vertex to forehead. As if pieces of the parietal bone were being torn from the head. As if something fell forword in occiput. There is aversion to milk, and milk <; the child has diarrhoea every time it nurses. Craving for acid drinks and fruits especially *apples*. but all <: > Lying down and *stretching* – compelled to stretch. The navel is a centre of many pains. The groins are strongly affected and the pelvic bones.

(A group of torpical diseases, Kala-Azar, Oriental Sore and Espundia, caused by infection with the *Leishmania donovani* parasite, have recently been brought within the therapeutic sphcre of preparations of *Antimony*. Other names for Kala-Azar are "Dum-dum fever" and Tropical splenomegaly". The disease sets in with rigor, or vomiting or both. The fever is irregular and remittent. The spleen becomes immensely large and the abdomen protuberant. Haemorrhages, diarrhoea and dysentery are complications, and death is by exhaustion. The treatment by *Ant. t.* is eminently successful, and the symptom correspondence is not difficult to trace. The administration usually adopted is by intravenous or intramuscular injection. The preparations recommended (*see* Tropical Diseases, by the Drs. Neatby) are (1) *Sodium antimonyl tartrate* (sodium taking the place of the potassium of *Antim, tart.*) 2 per cent solution, a dose containing 1-2 grain of the salt is injected every second or every third day working up to a maximum dose of 1 3-4 grains. The treatment is continued for two months after the fever has ceased. (2) *Stibacetin (Acetyl-p-aminophenyl stibiate of sodium) this is less poisonous, and can be given in doses of 0.1 gramme (1.54 grain) and working up to 0.8 gramme (12.3 grain).* (3) *Colloidal antimony sulphide* in an 0.2 c.c suspension in doses up to 20 c.c, amounting in all to 2 grammes of the drug. (4) For intramuscular injection *Antimony oxide,* in Martindale's formula one fiftieth grain of *Ant. oxide* in fifteen drops of glycerine and fifteen drops of distilled water).

Relations - It *antidotes* effects of alcohol. *Antidoted by* Morphia. Compare winter coughs in old people, *Ammc.* - but with *Ammc.* sputum is yellow. Aversion of, and < by milk *Na. c.* Recurrent rattling colds, *K. sul.* (*K. sul.* has not the pallid prostrations of *Ant. t.* patients). Catarrh, *Ant. c.* (wants the copious flows of mucus from inflamed membrane, and the passive state of *Ant. t.*). Headache in cold, *Ars.* Headache on waking in night, *Ant. s. a.* < *Causation* - Sun. Alcohol. Asphyxia. Drowning.

SYMPTOMS.

1. **MIND**

    Delirium with pleasurable expression.-
    (Suicidal mood; he raves and does not know what he is doing).
    Talks to himself.-
    Despairs of recovery.-
    Anxiety increases with the nausea.-
    Anxiety; with restlessness; during the paroxysm; with oppression on the chest.-
    Frightened at every trifle.-
    Apprehensive; with fulness about the heart and increased warmth; with restlessness.
    Dreads to be alone, even for a few moments, lest he should be dreadfully nervous and not know what to do with himself.
    Morose, dejected and sad, 4:30 p.m.
    Weeps if looked at.
    Crying with the cough.
    Pitiful whining before the attacks. (Infantile catarrh).
    Child cries on attempting to take the breast.
    Child clings to nurse and calls for help with cough.
    Unusual wild gaiety, towards evening, giving place to fretfulness and peevishness.
    Stupefaction and somnolence with numbness of head.
    Stupid and sleepy.
    Dullness of mind, imbecility.
    Apathy and indifference; even death would have been welcome.
    Desire to bite.
    The children get angry, weep and cry (whooping-cough).
    Cough aggravated when angry.
    Strong emotion followed by amblyopia (during pregnancy).

2. **HEAD**

    Giddy and sick.
    Vertigo alternating with drowsiness.
    Vertigo; on closing eyes; on walking; when raising head; must lie down, with nausea.
    Vertigo and violent chills running through the body with a sudden shock.

Fainting: with sweat on forehead; after a cold feeling in scrobiculus, followed by sleep.
Asphyxia from drowning.
Headache with sensitiveness in epigastrium.
Heat in the head, aggravated by motion.
Frequent risings of heat in the head, with thirst.
Forehead covered with cold sweat; head cold.
Heat on forehead without sweat, morning.
On coughing, heat and sweat on forehead, so that she became very dizzy.
Fine burning on frontal bone above r. temple.
Head heavy, can scarcely be held upright; must be supported behind.
Headache as from a band compressing forehead.
Inward boring into frontal bone between l. root of nose and eyebrow.
Heavy pain in forehead like waves, increasing and decreasing.
Pressive tensive pain, esp. in forehead, immediately after waking, ameliorated by cold water.
Tensive pain in forehead aggravated in the evening; after eating, and sitting bent; ameliorated by sitting up, lying high and in the cold.
Pressive sticking in forehead extends down into l. eye. with great desire to close the eyes. On waking in the night always has the same bad headache as if the brain were balled into a heavy lump only in l. half of forehead.
Tensive headache as if the hairs were put together in lumps.
Painful drawing in r. temple extends down to the zygoma and upper jaw.
Tension and sensitive pressure on vertex.
In afternoon, on motion, a surging from the neck upwards, over vertex towards forehead: with stupefaction and confusion of the senses, on standing for one minute.
Intermittent tearings in r. side of head.
Tearing in r. side of head and esp. deep in r. ear, on raising head after stooping.
On stooping severe violent stitches in l. parietal bone extending forward.
Violent sticking tearing from posterior portion of l. parietal bone to a place in front of vertex, that it seems as though a piece were being torn from the head, deep within, on standing, 8 a.m.; recurred next day at same hour.

Occiput becomes heavy, and an anxious oppressive sensation sets in.
Sensation in occiput on stooping as if something fell forward.
Raging and throbbing on r. side occiput, like ulceration, on rest and motion.
Scalp so sensitive can hardly bear the comb. [*Tinea. Plica polonica* (Hg.)]

3. EYES

Squinting.
Bloodshot.
Sclerotica yellow.
Must press lids tightly together.
Dull pressure over nose and one eye.
Violent tearing between root of nose and one eyebrow, as if someone took hold of her there by the skin; is painful and long lasting.
Vanishing of sight; and hearing.
Flickering before the eyes, aggravated by rising from sitting.

4. EARS

Twitching tearing in r. concha, evening, lying down disappearing in bed; morning, second day.
Ulcerative pain in r. concha, evening.
(sensation as if spectacle bows were pressing behind ears. Cured, J.H.C.)
Roaring in ear.
Fluttering over l. ear, as from a large bird; at same time a warmth passes to this ear, as if she stood near a hot stove.

5. NOSE

Stupefying tension across root of nose as if laced with a band.
Sensation over bridge of nose as though a horse-hair drawn tightly across it (cured in a case of sunstroke. J.H.C.)
A tearing and crawling in l. nostril as if sudden irritation to sneeze, which, however, does not occur.
Corners of nostrils ulcerated and painful.

6. FACE

Cold sweat on face; livid, expression of great suffering. Convulsive twitches in almost every muscle of face.
Countenance distorted with peculiar tetanic spasm of jaws as though endeavouring to bite everything within reach.
Incessant quivering of chin and lower jaw (cured. J.H.C.)

Tearing pain in whole side of face, even head and neck of that side.
Itching vesicles, upper and lower lips.
Burning r. side chin as from hot coal.
Drawing from chin along r. side lower jaw.
Dislocation of jaw; it remains open for a while after yawning.

7. TEETH

During dentition catarrhal hyperaemia (Hg).

8. MOUTH

Tongue painful or difficult to move about.
Tearing on l. side behind root of tongue, on swallowing.
Morning after rising mouth so sore can scarcely swallow, with white tongue and sour taste.
Unpleasant sensation on palate.
On posterior part of palate, sore sensation, and as if a hard body lay against it; without swallowing; ameliorated by eating bread (8 a.m.)
Speech difficult.

9. THROAT

Increased mucus secretion.
Sharp pain at throat.
Choking sensation.
Roughness in throat, with sensation *as if a small lump obstructed windpipe,* on hawking;
Throat *raw; swallowing difficult and painful.*
Soft palate and pharynx is red, covered with vesicles; many are opened, swollen, and covered with mucus..
Itching and dryness in throat which provokes hacking (morning).
Rapid swelling of tonsils and cervical glands.
Oesophagus sensitive, unchewed masses = much pain.

10. APPETITE

Though food tastes good and he has some appetite, yet he can only gradually get some food into his stomach, from which he feels better, and is relieved by pressure on abdomen.
Eats at noon with appetite, but after he is satisfied a kind of nausea attacks him at times.
Extraordinary appetite for apples.

Child eats little but drinks much.
Thirst constant and insatiable.
Drinks little and often.
Aversion to milk.
Disgust for whisky.
Thirst for beer and sour milk, with dryness in throat.
Desire for acids.
ABSENCE OF THIRST; THE WHOLE DAY.
After eating: cough with vomiting of food and mucus; sleeps; discomfort; toothache; nausea; pressure in stomach; backache; vomiting immediately; fever.
Aggravated after warm drinks, esp. milk.

11. STOMACH

Belching which ameliorates.
Eructations with gagging.
NAUSEA = GREAT ANXIETY.
Nausea and vomiting of curdled milk.
Vomiting till he becomes faint.
Waterbrash.
Nausea, then yawning with profuse lachrymation, followed by vomiting.
Vomits food and drink, even before the cough (in whooping cough).
Vomits tenacious mucus.
Vomits great masses of phlegm.
VOMITS WITH GREAT EFFORT.
Vomited matter tinged with blood; bloody, foamy fluid; bloody mucus.
Vomiting, in any position, except lying or r. side.
Vomiting with headache and trembling of hands.
Vomits then sleeps; vomiting returns after sleep.
Heaviness in stomach.
Craving sensation at stomach.
Emptiness in stomach.
At night sensation as if stomach loaded.
Weight at stomach, ameliorated by open air, aggravated in room.
Violent pains at epigastrium which was tense.
Cramps in stomach.
Whirling in pit of stomach with rapid action of heart; which threatens to rupture heart.
Feeling as of cold water at pit of stomach, with it he feels faint, falls down; then heat in head.

Addition to Classical Materia Medica 25

Burning heat in stomach.
Warmth in stomach followed by violent pain in forehead and back of throat.

12. ABDOMEN

Liver increased in size.
Liver sensitive to contact.
Pressure in hypochondria with distention, aggravated in region of liver.
Jaundice with pneumonia, esp. r.
Meteorism.
Warmth about navel, gradually extending over whole abdomen.
Colic around nevel, early morning.
Pains in abdomen, after eating; after vomiting.
Violent pressive tension in abdomen, esp. over bladder.
Violent pain at epigastrium and through whole abdomen, with constant spasmodic contractions of abdominal muscles.
Cutting in abdomen; and across lower abdomen it lies like a stone, with great nausea; after six ineffectual retchings followed by ineffecutal efforts at stool, vomiting with great exertion, trembling in abdomen, and bending together, then two diarrhoeic stools.
Stitches.
Warmth in lower abdomen, as if had drunk something very warm; it wanders about and finally up to stomach.
Tensive drawing towards bladder.
Wakes 1 a.m. with gripes above pubis and icy coldness of whole body; cold sweat breaks out in profusion; intense heat.
Spasmodic drawing from thigh to abdomen.
Pressure in hypogastrium and aching, with cold shivers, as if menses whould appear.
Stitches over pubis.
Very violent burning soreness in r. groin.
Rheumatic pain in l. pelvic bone.
Violent twisting *cutting pains tearing from hypogastrium down thighs to knees like labour pains.*
Pains in groins and cold creeps before menses.
Painful sensation in hypogastrium = intense mental restlessness and aversion to work.
Sensitiveness of abdomen.
Tetanic rigidity of abdominal muscles, extending to legs and then to upper extremities.

13. STOOLS AND ANUS

   Sudden, violent, alarming stitch, from lower abdomen down through rectum.
   Involuntary evacuation of much mucus with dead roundworms.
   Involuntary watery blood-streaked stools.
   Uncommonly hard stool-difficult to pass.
   Stools green as grass, slimy.
   Watery, sometimes slimy and greenish diarrhoea, aggravated each time child nurses.
   Diarrhoea slimy, yeast-like, of cadaverous smell.

14. URINARY ORGANS

   Violent tension in perineum, upon walking, with strong desire to urinate.
   Violent burning in urethra, during and after urinating.
   The urging to urinate and burning in urethra increase, only a little urine passes; the last drops are bloody and accompanied by violent pains in bladder.

15. MALE SEXUAL ORGANS

   Buring tickling irritation extends from rectum through urethra to glans where it is most severe.
   Pustles on genitals and thighs.

16. FEMALE SEXUAL ORGANS

   Severe bearing down in vagina.
   Menses six days too early, weak, but only two days.
   Before menses: pains in groins and cold creeping.
   During pregnancy: gastric derangements; vomiting of mucus; salivation; nausea and faintness; amblyopia after strong emotions.
   Puerperal convulsions, great jactitation of muscles.
   Asphyxia neonatorum.

17. RESPIRATORY ORGANS

   Excretion of tough mucus.
   Voice small and changed.
   Hoarsensess; aggravated on talking; morning.
   Cough and yawning consecutively.
   Cough after eating, vomits food and mucus.
   Child grasps larynx with cough.
   Catarrh provokes cough, *though she had no power to cough.*
   Croup with inability to swallow.

Addition to Classical Materia Medica   27

Obvious paralysis in croup (Hg.)
Unequal breathing, now shorter then longer, much more frequent lying down, ameliorated when carried sitting upright.
Gasps for air at beginning of every coughing spell.
Impending paralysis of lungs.
Atelectasis-Relieves death-rattle (Hg.)
Cough with much rattling in chest and no expectoration.
Every cough causes unbearable pains in the chest.
Coughing with crying; or dozing; or twitching of the face.
Thick bloody sputa.
Sputa foaming, mixed with blood.

18. **CHEST**

Full feeling in chest.
Pain r. side, behind and at base of chest aggravated by deep breathing.
Stitches in l. upper chest and l. axilla.
Burning in l. breast, near shoulder, more externally aggravated by pressing or rubbing.
Itching stitch on r. nipple.
Crawling as of insects above l. mamma.
Stitches in l. breast with cough.

19. **HEART**

So warm about the heart she must let the arms sink down with general weakness.
Pressure or heaviness in praecordium.

20. **NECK AND BACK**

Cramp in neck muscles.
Pressive sense of fatigue in neck muscles, close to occiput, esp. r. side.
Dose not like anything to touch him; inclination to unbutton shirt collar.
On turning neck, painful aching over the l. scapula, comes suddenly 24 hours later over the r. scapula.
Pain like fatigue in back aggravated after eating and *while sitting.*
Pains in small of back, before and on rising from bed, as if one carried a weight there; ameliorated after rising.
Short, sticking, tearing pain, esp. in lower r. side of back, near r. hip.

21. **LIMBS**

    Insensibility and coldness of limbs. R. arm and hand and both great toes cold to touch. Burning, tearing and drawing in joints.

22. **UPPER LIMBS**

    Frequent twitching of the tendons in arms and hands.
    Pain as of dislocation in r. shoulder.
    Violent tearing externally in r. shoulder, followed by itching.
    Violent itching in l. shoulder a number of vesicles arise, must scratch till they bleed, without relief to itching, where upon the spot burns.
    Stitching and twinging below l. axilla; then a stitch with twinging in condyles of l. elbow.
    Burning in r. humerus as if in the marrow. Burning inside surface r. upper arm; with yawning.
    Eruptions like itch on forearm near wrist.
    Hands cold and moist.
    On coughing, heat and moisture of hands and sweat of head.
    On back of l. hand, on touching the hairs, fine severe stitches.
    When she wants to clench her first, or extend her fingers, they are tense as if swollen.
    Fingers firmly contracted, every muscle in extraordinary state of rigidity.
    Violent itching of palm.

23. **LOWER LIMBS**

    On each buttock there are four tensively painful pimples which pain like a boil on pressure.
    Numbness and coldness in the legs.
    Spasmodic twitchings in muscles of thigh.
    Outward stitching in varices.
    Slight swelling and stiffness on malleoli of r. foot.
    Soreness between little and next toe of r. foot.

24. **GENERALITIES**

    Constant contractions of all the muscles esp. of abdomen and upper extremities.
    Tetanus.

Excessive restlessness.
Condition like intoxication.
Faintness
Syncope.

25. SKIN

Shrivelled, dry.
Wilted; cool; as if dead.
Dry and burning hot on chest and hands, cool on feet.
Eruption fails to appear and convulsions set in.

26. SLEEP

Great sleepiness, if he sits still he sleeps immediately, with vivid dreams of a continuation of his previous thoughts.
He had scarcely fallen asleep when he was seized with electric shocks and jerks, all of which came from the abdomen; it threw now one arm, now arm, now another away from his body; now a foot; now it threw the whole body into the air.
Dreams of fire.

[From the HOMOEOPATHIC RECORDER, August 1929 *Pages 564 – 573*]